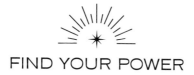

FIND YOUR POWER

MINDFULNESS

An Hachette UK Company
www.hachette.co.uk

First published in Great Britain in 2023 by Godsfield,
an imprint of Octopus Publishing Group Ltd
Carmelite House, 50 Victoria Embankment, London EC4Y 0DZ
www.octopusbooks.co.uk

ISBN 978-1-8418-1555-8

A CIP catalogue record for this book is available from the British Library

Printed and bound in China

10 9 8 7 6 5 4 3 2 1

Publisher: Lucy Pessell
Designer: Isobel Platt
Editor: Feyi Oyesanya
Assistant Editor: Samina Rahman
Production Controller: Allison Gonsalves

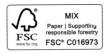

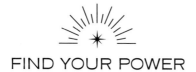

FIND YOUR POWER

MINDFULNESS

ALINA CURTIS

GODSFIELD

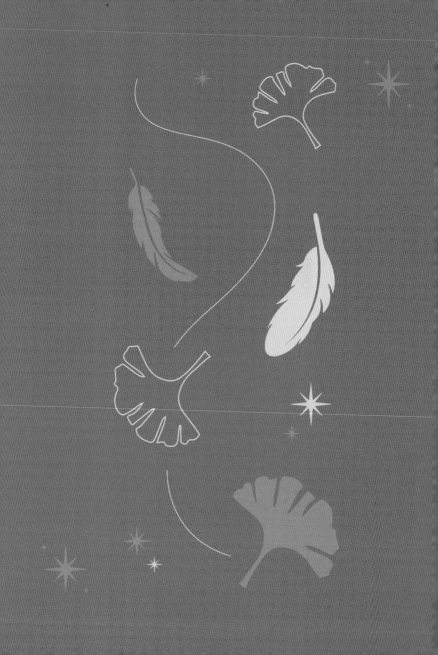

CONTENTS

FIND
YOUR
POWER

When daily life becomes busy and your time and energy is pulled in many different directions, it can be difficult to find time to nourish yourself. Prioritizing your own wellbeing can be a struggle and you risk feeling overwhelmed, unsure of where to turn and what you need in order to feel lighter and find your inner strength.

Taking some time to focus on yourself, answering questions you may be avoiding or facing problems that are simmering away under the surface is the best gift you can give yourself. But it can be difficult to know where to start.

Sometimes all you need to learn life's big lessons is a little guidance. In this series of books you will learn about personal healing, self-empowerment and how to nourish your spirit. Explore practices which will help you to get clear on what you really want, and that will encourage you to acknowledge – and deal with – any limiting beliefs or negative thoughts that might be holding you back in living life to your fullest power.

These books provide invaluable advice on how to create the best conditions for a healthier, happier, and more fulfilled life. Bursting with essential background, revealing insights and useful activities and exercises to enable you to understand and expand your personal practices every day, it's time to delve into your spiritual journey and truly Find Your Power.

Other titles in the series:

- *Find Your Power: Tarot*
- *Find Your Power: Manifest*
- *Find Your Power: Numerology*
- *Find Your Power: Runes*
- *Find Your Power: Crystals*
- *Find Your Power: Chakra*
- *Find Your Power: Meditation*

INTRODUCTION

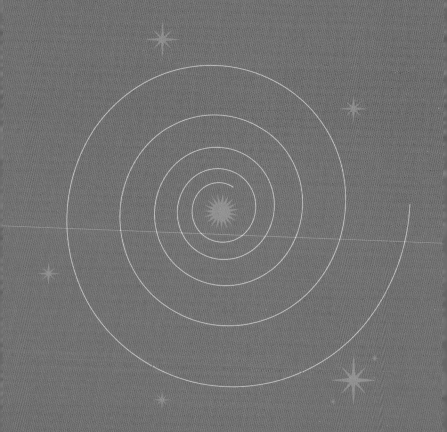

There are days when everything seems like a blur.

The modern world can be a whirlwind of distractions and noise. Our phones buzz with notifications, our screens fill with suggested videos, our inboxes flood with emails. And with each buzz and ping and distraction, we are pulled away from whatever it is we are doing. Our minds are fractured, split between multiple things. We eat in front of the TV, without fully noticing the food or what we're watching. We scroll on our phones while having coffee with friends; we walk to and from work with our headphones in, our minds partly on the commute and partly on the podcast – and partly on everything we have to do that day.

We tell ourselves we are multitasking; we tell ourselves we are busy. We tell ourselves we just don't have time.

Now think for a moment.

What did you have for dinner last night?

How did the first mouthful taste? What was the texture like, the fragrance, the temperature?

What was your shower like this morning?

How did the water feel on your back? What did your shampoo smell like? How did the towel feel afterwards, when you stepped out of the shower and wrapped it around you?

It's OK if you can't remember. Most of us can't. But what if we tried to experience everything a little more carefully, a little more in the moment?

A little more *mindfully*?

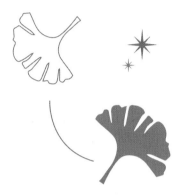

Mindfulness is an indispensable tool for daily living. It helps us to cultivate a clear and comprehensive awareness of where we are and what is happening within and around us, without allowing the mind to wander.

By living mindfully, we develop a fresh relationship with all our everyday activities, from brushing our teeth, to engaging in work, or making love. Practising mindfulness awakens us to a liberated life and the experience of natural joy day to day. It keeps us connected to and in tune with the world around us and ourselves.

Through the power of mindfulness, we recognize that the here and now can be a vehicle leading to profound understanding.

The practice of mindfulness can be traced back to meditation techniques practised in a number of Buddhist and Hindu traditions, but we do not have to have any particular religious beliefs to practise and benefit from mindfulness; anyone can experience the powerful impact it can have on their daily existence.

The more we practise, the more we realize that mindfulness is a simple and readily available resource for the young and old, the healthy and sick, the successful and unsuccessful. Each of us can benefit from mindful living and the practices that support it.

If we commit ourselves to the practice of mindful living, we experience countless benefits. We develop respect, care and appreciation for our place in this world. We become calmer and find it easier to concentrate. We experience the here and now in ever deepening ways. Through our developing powers of observation, we see things more clearly and are able to respond to different situations from a place of clarity.

Mindfulness helps us become better able to cope with the frustrations of everyday life, from stressful situations at work to challenging family dynamics. It can help us develop our sense of compassion and kindness, and learn how to become more patient with others. It can teach us how to navigate difficult situations rather than simply avoiding them, and how to find moments of peace in a world that seems full of chaos.

Through the practice of mindfulness, we can deepen our harmonious relationship with

✳

Practising mindfulness awakens us to a liberated life and the experience of natural joy day to day.

✳

✳

Mindfulness is permission to truly experience what you are feeling, without attachment to those feelings.

✳

daily life and learn to love the challenge of working with the ordinary and the everyday.

There are hundreds of opportunities to practise mindfulness throughout our days, from drinking tea to waiting for the bus – and with each opportunity we take, we learn to appreciate our lives in a new way, moment by moment.

It's a common misunderstanding that mindfulness is simply about happiness. You may have visions of a person sitting in meditation with an expression of sheer bliss on their face. However, the truth is that although mindfulness can help you to uncover a more joyful and peaceful life, there's a lot more to it than that.

Mindfulness will certainly heighten your awareness when you do experience happiness, but it will also bring your attention to so much more. Mindfulness is permission to truly experience

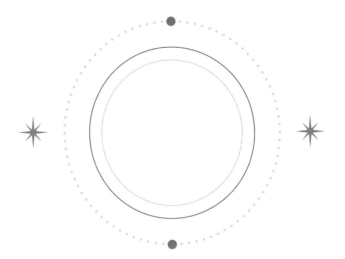

what you are feeling, without attachment to those feelings.

As you develop your mindfulness practice, you might experience sadness or frustration or longing. The key is to allow yourself to notice, experience and investigate the thoughts or emotions that ask for your attention, without becoming those thoughts or emotions.

You are not your thoughts. Thoughts come into the mind.

They can be very powerful, and it can be tempting to claim those thoughts as a set belief or a fact – I am shy, I don't cry – but nothing is set. Nothing is permanent. Notice the feeling, feel it, but don't take ownership of it. Instead of I am shy, allow yourself to think, I am experiencing a feeling of shyness in this moment. In this way, you notice the thought, and perhaps even examine it, but you do not hold on to it or define yourself by it.

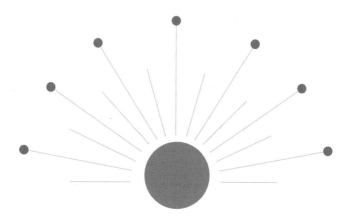

In practising mindfulness, you are taking a step towards truly accepting what is. When we are in acceptance, we are no longer gripped by overpowering thoughts or emotions. This is not to say that we don't experience them, but that when we do, we are able to recognize them for what they are.

In this book, we will explore mindfulness by looking at four of the key things it can bring to your life:

Intention: A sense of purpose and deliberateness in all that you do.

Presence: A sense of inhabiting your physical body and its place in the world, and of being in the moment.

Clarity: A sense of calmness, understanding and awareness of yourself and the world around you.

Connection: A sense of how everything ties together, from the natural world to the relationships you have with others.

Each chapter will include exercises and ideas to help you build elements of mindfulness into your life in a way that works for you. These exercises will encourage you to take action to understand and connect with the ideas we will be exploring. They might include meditations, activities or challenges. Use these exercises as an opportunity to take time out of your day to focus on mindfulness and discover how it can help you find clarity and focus.

JOURNAL PROMPTS

There will also be journaling prompts to help you dive more deeply into the elements of mindfulness that really resonate with you. These prompts will invite you to explore these ideas more closely by writing about them. If you find this practice useful, try to incorporate the act of journaling more regularly into your daily life. It is a valuable mindfulness practice.

When we are in acceptance, we are no longer gripped by overpowering thoughts.

JOURNALING

Journaling is an opportunity for self-enquiry and exploration. It is just you, your thoughts and feelings, and a notebook. There is so much potential in this simplicity. You are giving yourself permission to be present with yourself, to open up your senses and to listen to the whispers from within.

Writing mindfully for just a few minutes each day is a wonderful practice that can help bring you into the present moment. It encourages you to notice your own presence and how you are feeling right now in your body and mind. It also encourages you to notice and be engaged with the richness of life in all its detail. Whether you are experiencing pure joy or pure heartache, it is all part of your experience of life.

Writing something down enables you to process it. Old thoughts or emotions that have become stuck or held too tightly are given acknowledgement and can then be released to make space for new manifestations or dreams. Putting pen to paper can help you to work through and let go of the emotional baggage of the day, as well as bigger things, like deeply rooted self-limiting beliefs and unhelpful thought patterns.

Journaling can also be a really useful tool for practising gratitude (see page 107). It's amazing how many things for which you are grateful can be expressed on paper in just five minutes – or one minute. It can also be a powerful way to reinforce and remind yourself of all the resources you carry with you each day, from your sense of humour and your intelligence to the things you know help to relax or nourish you.

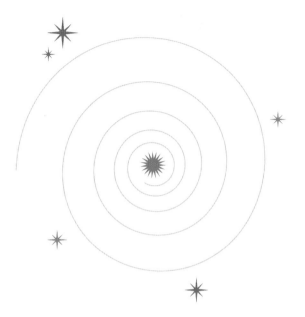

And because writing and other creative activities put your mind into a meditative or 'theta' state, journaling can even help to rewire your brain. A calmer mind copes more easily with stressful situations and makes decisions more effectively.

Through regular journaling and mindful self-reflection, you develop the ability to spot your habits and behaviour patterns, and this awareness helps you to make changes where they are needed.

Writing also sharpens your powers of observation, so that you can live each day with increased awareness of your connections with others and the world around you, bringing clarity to each moment.

When you notice the details of life, is it like a flower that blossoms.

INTENTION

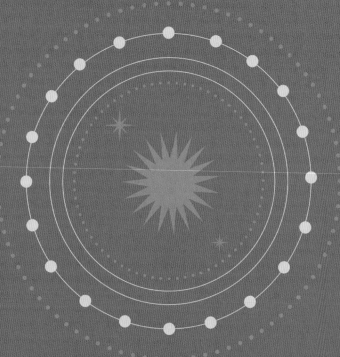

The next thing you do,
do it on purpose.

Because we are busy, because
we are distracted, because we
are stressed, we often do things
in a hurry, sometimes carelessly,
sometimes without even noticing
we're doing them. We quickly
hang out the laundry when the
washing machine beeps, but our
thoughts are on that big meeting
tomorrow, or the TV show we're
watching out of the corner of our
eyes, and we rush through the task,
sometimes not even hanging things
up with care so they don't dry as
quickly. We remember a friend's
birthday is coming up, so we
hurriedly order them a gift online,
our minds already rushing ahead
to the next item on the to-do list
– only to realize that in our haste,
we've entered the wrong delivery
address, and now need to email the
seller and try to unpick the mess.

What if, instead, we hung out our
laundry with care, one piece at
a time, taking the time to notice
the smell of the clean linen?
What if, as we selected our
friend's gift, we thought about
that friend, how much we care
about them, how pleased we are
to be celebrating their birthday?

Of course, very few of us have
time to carry out every single
daily task at a glacial pace, but
even just changing our attitudes
and paying a little more attention
can help us to move through
the world – and our lives – with
more purpose and intention.

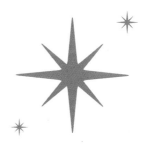

Leave your phone somewhere else; don't go and sit at your laptop or start checking emails.

A CUP OF TEA

We'll begin with tea. It seems as good a place as any.

Have you ever been camping? When camping in the outdoors, we are reminded of the true wonder of that first morning cup of tea – waiting for the water to boil over the stove or the fire, warming your hands around the cup, and watching the steam rise as the sun begins to peek over the horizon. It's a genuinely special experience.

Making a cup of tea before going to work in the morning may not seem to have the same romantic symbolism, but by granting it the appreciation and attention you'd give to that magical campfire cuppa, you can create a quiet and rather beautiful moment in your morning routine.

Take a few minutes to sit with your first cup of tea of the day. Try to find a peaceful corner. Leave your phone somewhere else; don't go and sit at your laptop or start checking emails. Just sit with your tea.

Feel the warmth of the cup. Notice the steam rising and the aroma of the liquid. Lift it to your lips and take the first sip. Feel the warmth of it on your tongue, in your throat. Savour it and feel grateful for it.

Taking these moments in the morning with your tea (or coffee, if you prefer!) will create a sense of stillness that you can hold with you throughout the ups and downs of a busy day.

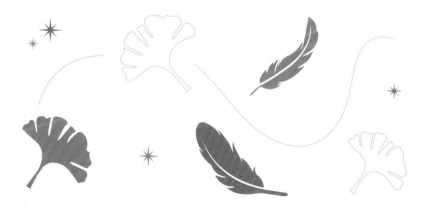

BREATH

Mindfulness starts with the breath.

Every breath we take confirms our moment-to-moment relationship with the world. Setting aside even a few minutes every day to breathe with mindful awareness can contribute so much to our emotional, mental and spiritual wellbeing. Breathing deeply, whether through exercise or intention, is important for the body, since full breaths nourish the cells more completely. It also encourages us to slow down, and when we slow down, we become mindful.

'For breath is life, and if you breathe well, you will live long on earth.'

Sanskrit proverb

THE BENEFITS OF MINDFUL BREATHING

As we cultivate greater mindfulness of breathing, we begin to experience its many benefits.

Mindful breathing helps us to achieve:

- calmness and concentration
- the feeling of being centred
- harmony of body and mind

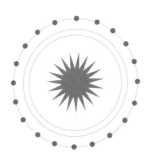

- the ability to stay steady in stressful or threatening situations

- deep joy and inner contentment

- the capacity to clear the mind of excessive thinking

- a deep sense of intimacy and connection with organic life

- an experience of inner freedom in the midst of unfolding events

As we mindfully breathe in and out, even for a few minutes, we have the chance to relax and to cut through much that is false within – projections, daydreams, fantasies, mind games and mental wanderings. As we gain the ability to see through our illusions, we discover for ourselves what is valid, true and relevant.

✳

Every breath we take confirms our moment-to-moment relationship with the world.

✳

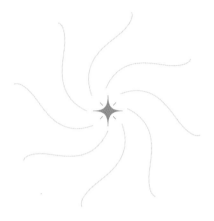

> **As we develop mindfulness of breathing, we settle into the present until we feel at home with what is.**

Since the breath is always with us, always valid and relevant to our lives, focusing on it helps to teach us to distinguish between truth and illusion, clarity and confusion, valid perception and illusory projection. As we practise this skill, we find it easier to avoid conflict and inner turmoil, as well as the problems we cause for others when we confuse fact and fantasy. As we develop mindfulness of breathing, we settle into the present until we feel at home with what is.

But how do we achieve this?

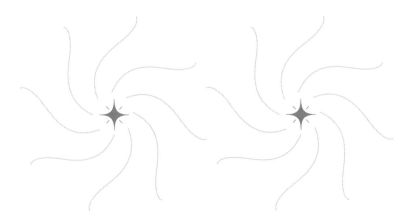

FOCUSING ON THE BREATH

There are several techniques for focusing on the breath.

You might choose to observe the breath by focusing your attention on the spot above your upper lip, where the air enters or leaves through your nostrils. If you prefer, you can observe the rise and fall of the chest, or the rise and fall of the abdomen, during the cycle of each inhalation and exhalation.

Alternatively, you can try to be aware of the whole process of the breath from start to finish. If you are just getting started with a mindfulness of breathing practice, try to be aware of the whole breath from the time the air travels up through your nose and down into your lungs, to the final exhalation.

MINDFUL BREATHING

When the mind feels troubled, breathe in and breathe out deeply. You can do this anywhere. You can even do it at work, although you might want to try and find a quiet space so you can focus. As you become more used to mindful breathing, you can even do it as you walk along.

As you do this practice, pay particular attention to the out-breath, and try to relax into it.

1. Sit somewhere quiet where you can be alone for a few minutes. Your eyes can be open or closed.

2. Breathe. Make the breath a little longer and deeper than usual for the first two or three minutes so that you can experience the expansion of your body as the oxygen enters, and the sense of settling down as your body expels the carbon dioxide. Try to experience your breaths as closely as possible during this period, following them through your body. Remember that the mind most easily wanders on the out-breath.

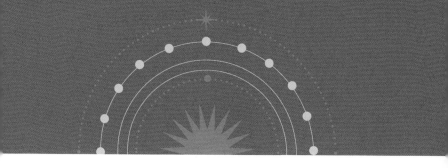

3. If your mind does wander, don't get frustrated with yourself. Just notice the distraction, and try to let it drift away.

4. When you're finished, try to hold on to this sense of calm, focus and intentional breathing.

When we sit calmly and bring mindfulness to the breath, we flood the body with life energy from head to toe. You can use this powerful technique in many situations.

If you feel yourself holding back unnecessarily from a situation, for example speaking up in a meeting or sharing an idea, then take a few moments to breathe through any fear you might be feeling, and then act.

If somebody is saying unkind words to you, mindfully breathe in and out rather than reacting. Don't give others authority over your state of mind.

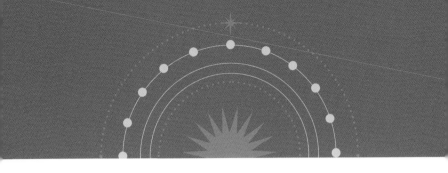

Journal prompt: Let something go

One of the ways in which mindfulness can help us bring intention into our lives is not just what we choose to focus on, but what we choose to let go.

If we're not careful, it's easy to find ourselves carrying a great deal of emotional and mental baggage around with us throughout our days: old stories, hurts, patterns of behaviour, beliefs about ourselves and preconceptions about others. No wonder we often feel laden down, as if we're carrying more with us than we can handle.

Think about some of the things you are carrying with you that are weighing you down and don't serve you. Begin to write them down in your journal. As you write, imagine that you are putting these things down, letting them go. Sense how much lighter and freer you feel.

What can you let go of today?

SPEAK WITH INTENTION

Speech is one of the ways in which we communicate most with others. Being able to connect verbally and express ourselves through language is a gift, but we often fail to appreciate it – and sometimes we even misuse it.

Try to practise speaking with intention and mindfulness, thinking about what you want to say and how you want to express it. Instead of wasting words on idly complaining, repeating gossip or saying something unkind, try to start each day with a commitment to letting go of the impulse to use unwise speech.

Aim to make your speech unhurried, calm and thoughtful, even in the face of provocation. By resisting idle chatter and unkind speech, we can move towards communicating in a way that feels mindful, intentional and useful.

'Be like a tree and let the dead leaves drop.'

Rumi

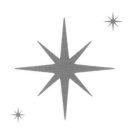

TAKE A CLOSER LOOK

Choose an object that features regularly in your everyday life. It could be a house key, a ring, a pen – something fairly small, that you use or see so often that you barely even notice it.

Now – notice it.

Examine it in great detail. What does it look like? How does it feel in your hand? Think about its weight, its texture, its shape. What is it made of? Does it have sharp or soft edges? Is there anything about it that you find beautiful?

Pay attention to your own feelings in response to noticing the object's details.

Now think about how many other objects just like this you interact with on a daily basis – without really noticing.

Make a commitment to notice them more often.

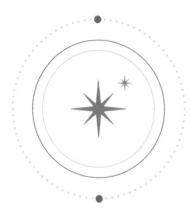

Patience is the capacity to stay steady and calm despite uncertainty. Through mindfulness practice and concentrating on the here and now, we learn to stay grounded in both the short and long term.

Without patience, we become adversely affected by what we hear, sense or think. We find our levels of agitation increasing through the desire for something to change more quickly than the circumstances allow.

This is something that is ever more noticeable in the modern world, where so much of our lives are geared towards speed and convenience. We are used to being able to order something online and having it delivered the next day, or being able watch the next episode of a TV show straight away on a streaming service rather than waiting for it to be broadcast next week. We can make a journey in a matter of hours that once would have taken days; if we need to speak to someone who is a hundred – or a thousand – miles away, we can be connected with them in seconds. These are exciting developments that can be very positive, but they can also limit our capacity for patience – and patience is essential if we are to live mindful, intentional lives.

DEVELOPING PATIENCE

- Be mindful that impatience easily shows itself in tone of voice, attitude and body language. Pay attention to these signals in yourself; try adjusting your posture or tone. Making a conscious effort to appear more patient can help you to actually feel that way too.

- Use breathing exercises to allow the cells in your body to relax.

- If you are in a long queue or stuck in a waiting room, try to use this as an opportunity to practise mindful patience. Instead of resisting the wait, dwelling on how infuriating it is or trying to distract yourself by playing on your phone, use the time to wait on purpose. Let waiting be the thing that you are doing. If feelings of stress or frustration arise, notice them, but do not hold on to them. Sit (or stand) and breathe. And wait.

- Develop steadfastness in the here and now by accepting it when things don't go to plan, rather than focusing on a sense of impatience. Acknowledge that feeling peaceful and calm is far preferable to being uptight when events do not go your way. Accepting a minor inconvenience rather than resisting something that is beyond your control can help you to stay calm and gain perspective.

- Remind yourself that your practice will help you to develop patience and inner peace. Acknowledge that you will experience setbacks. Keep practising for your own peace of mind as well as to take the pressure off others.

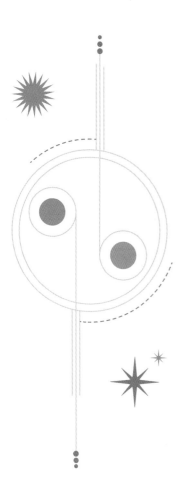

Be mindful that impatience easily shows itself in tone of voice, attitude and body language.

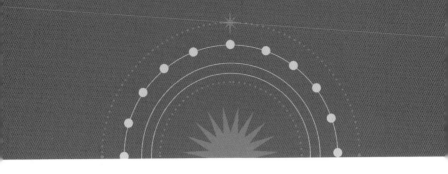

Journal prompt: The power of patience

If we become truly mindful of the impact of patience – or impatience, for that matter – it will lead to inner change, and to an understanding that life has its own movement, and can't just be bent to meet our demands.

1. In your journal, write out a list of the benefits of patience.

2. Reflect on the list and memorise two or three points. Endeavour to remember them, even in moments of brief impatience.

3. Think about the last time you were feeling impatient. How might the situation have played out differently if you had been able to practise mindful patience? Doing the washing-up isn't the most glamorous of tasks, but it's an important part of keeping our homes clean and comfortable to be in. Existing in a space that feels calm and orderly helps us to feel that way, too.

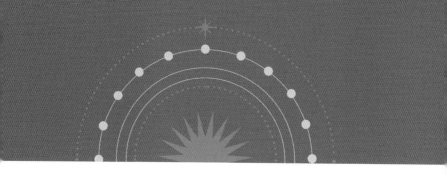

Next time you have to wash up after a meal, try to complete the job mindfully. Don't be tempted to put on a podcast or listen to music. Just be in the moment, doing what you are doing. Feel the water; notice the scent of the washing-up liquid and the shape of the bubbles.

Pick up each item with care and intention and focus your attention on it as you wash it. Consider the effort that went into making each item, and the many uses you get out of each one. If you become distracted and find your mind wandering, that's fine. Just try to come back to the present moment.

You may begin to find you get a sense of satisfaction out of a job well done and the feeling of taking care of your space and your belongings; you might even discover that you're enjoying yourself.

This approach can be applied to any number of household tasks that are usually considered dull, like folding laundry, putting away groceries, dusting or vacuuming.

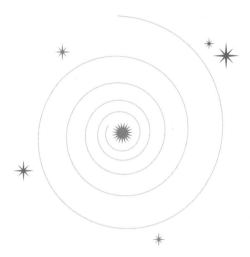

DO ONE THING AT A TIME

We've all been there. You're sitting at your desk with some reading material that you need to look through and review before a meeting this afternoon. You're just about to dive in when – ping! – an email pops up. It's a colleague, asking you to send over a report you've been working on. You just need to give it a quick edit before you send it. So, you open the document and start typing, but then your phone buzzes. It's a friend texting you about your plans for this evening. You decide you'll

respond to them later, but now your phone is in your hand, so you take a quick look at social media. Someone's posted a picture of the coffee they had this morning, and that reminds you that you haven't had your coffee yet. So you decide to go and get one from the canteen – and then you'll finish the report, reply to your friend, review the reading material for the meeting...

Being able to juggle different tasks and manage a changing workflow is an important part of many jobs today, but the rise of emails, instant chat and constant connectivity means that sometimes we're not so much juggling as dropping ball after ball and diving for cover as still more rain down on us.

Try to do one thing at a time, and keep doing it until it's done. Do it with purpose and intention, and do it well. When you've finished, turn to the next task.

Of course, this won't always be possible – priorities change, and sometimes we have to go with the flow. But when it is within your control, embrace that control and focus on one task at a time. It will help you feel more focused and centred – and with your mind less scattered and your attention undivided, you'll get more done.

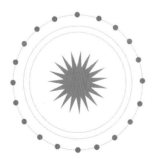

Try to do one thing at a time, and keep doing it until it's done.

EATING MINDFULLY

We rarely, if ever, focus entirely on the sensory stimulation of eating. We might be talking at the same time, or reading, working, watching television or scrolling on our phones. In fact, we're so used to doing something else at the same time as eating that it would probably feel strange to just...eat.

This is a practice that your digestion will thank you for, as studies have shown that the absorption of nutrients is increased when you eat mindfully.

Taking the time to notice and enjoy our food in this way brings us into a place of sensory awareness, which in turn helps us to be more aware of the details of life in general.

So the next time you eat a meal, try to do it with mindfulness and intention. Bring your awareness to the food on your plate: the colours, the aromas. Take a moment to feel gratitude for the food, and for all the hard work by various people that has brought it here. Consider the hours and days of labour in growing, harvesting, transporting and cooking each item on your plate. Doesn't it deserve your attention?

Take a mouthful – how does it taste? Salty, sweet, sour? Does it have a spicy heat to it, or is it cooling, like a cucumber? What is the texture like? Crisp, crunchy, smooth, creamy?

Mindful eating can also be a really useful practice if you are prone to stress-eating, or if you're trying to reduce your consumption of certain things, like processed foods or refined sugar. Practising a more mindful approach to eating means you are less likely to eat something without thinking, and can help you stick to healthier choices.

This isn't to say that mindful eating has to be all salads and carrot sticks, though! Imagine the sense of joyful indulgence you could experience by slowly and mindfully eating an ice cream sundae or a perfectly melty cheese toastie.

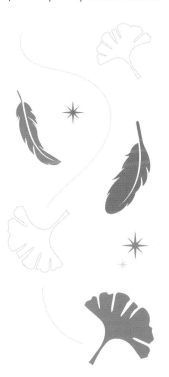

The next time you eat a meal, try to do it with mindfulness and intention. Bring your awareness to the food on your plate.

> The greatest contribution to a good night's sleep is a relaxed attitude towards events during the day.

A MINDFUL APPROACH TO SLEEP

Many people experience problems with sleep, whether they struggle with restless nights here and there, or find it distressingly difficult to get to sleep every evening. A lack of restful sleep affects our daily lives, and can leave us feeling tired, short-tempered and wiped out. Taking a mindful and intentional approach to sleep can make a real difference.

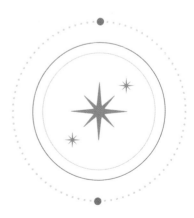

Practising mindfulness during the day, and considering the ideas outlined below, may help you to make a relaxed transition from the demands and stimulation of a busy day to a deep and peaceful sleep.

- Limit your intake of stimulants such as caffeine, tobacco and sugar, especially shortly before going to bed. Similarly, try to avoid screens and bright lights late in the evening.

- Avoid eating a heavy meal for at least two hours before bedtime. Instead, choose easily digestible, nutritious foods. Some foods, for example bananas and lettuce, are thought to have sleep-inducing properties.

- Try to create a calming and relaxing bedtime routine. Lower the lighting, wear comfortable pyjamas, and take your time with things like evening skincare and brushing your teeth. Use these routines as a way to prepare yourself physically and mentally for sleep, so that your mind and body can start to wind down in advance. As you repeat these routines, they will begin to signal to your mind that it is time for bed.

- We all know posture is important when we're sitting at our desks, but it's also something you should think about when you're in bed. Relax your whole body into the mattress. Lie there mindfully, quietly maximising the sense of rest. Consider also the position you sleep in and the kind of mattress you use. Experiment and see what works for you.

- The greatest contribution to a good night's sleep is a relaxed attitude towards events during the day – a mindful attitude during the day can make a huge difference when it comes to sleeping at night.

YOUR PRIORITIES

Journal prompt: What are your priorities?

Practising mindfulness and living with intention can help you to identify the things that really matter to you. Intention is like a seed; it is the commitment and the determination to act in a certain way, but it doesn't rely on any attachment to a specific outcome. After all, you cannot control the future, only how you act in this moment.

As you build your mindfulness practice, your intentions will become clearer; they will speak to you from within.

Think about one important area of your life: it could be your relationship, your career, your home, your goals for the future – whatever feels right to you. In your journal, write about your primary intentions in that area. Be totally honest.

Are you satisfied with these intentions? Do you want to change them?

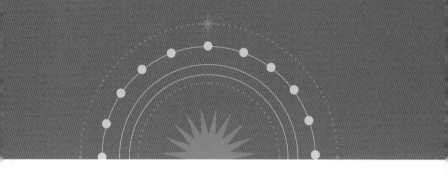

If you want to make changes to your intentions, be clear about these changes. Write them down and revisit this journal entry to remind yourself of them.

Remember that wisdom includes the application of skilful intention for the benefit of yourself and others.

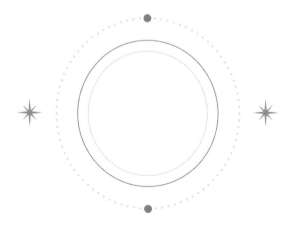

PRESENCE

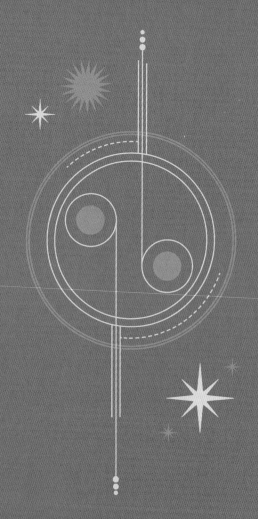

Be where you are.

The past is behind you,
the future lies ahead, and
life is truly experienced in
the present moment.

But because we live so much of our
lives remotely – talking to people
who aren't in the room with us,
watching footage of other places,
looking at a screen rather than
the scene in front of us – it's easy
to become disconnected from
where we are. Not just the space
we're in, but the bodies we're in.

Think about the last time you had
a cold: a sore throat, a blocked
nose, a headache. It's a wretched
feeling, and when we're ill, we
long to feel better, to be able to
breathe easily again. But when
we're well, we very rarely notice
our bodies. If they're doing
everything they're supposed to, we
don't really pay attention to them.

Making the effort to become
more mindfully present in your
body and the space you inhabit
can help you to slow down,
reconnect with yourself, and foster
a sense of wellbeing and calm.

HOW DO YOU FEEL?

How often do you reply 'Fine,'
to the question 'How are
you?', without even thinking
about your answer?

What if you stopped to think
about it? How are you, really?

Do you even know?

Are you cold, hot, tired, on edge,
at peace? Are you hungry? Are
you bored, frustrated, excited,
annoyed? Perhaps you feel a
little hollowed out and low after
a tough week, or energised and
eager for the day ahead?

However you feel, it's possible
– probable – that 'Fine' doesn't
really cover it.

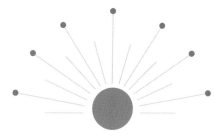

Mindfulness practices can help you really get in touch with how you feel, both physically and emotionally, and in so doing can help you develop a sense of presence.

FOCUS ON THE SENSES

One of the easiest and most natural ways to feel present in your body is to focus on your senses: really connecting with that experience, drawing close to it and savouring it for a few moments. Adopting this practice will heighten your awareness of the rich details of everyday life, and remind you of all those sensory moments that bring you joy or wake you up.

SMELL

Smell can be deeply evocative – catching a hint of a stranger's perfume in a crowded space can remind us of someone we haven't spoken to for years; taking a moment to sniff a ruby-red ripe tomato can transport us to a beloved grandparent's greenhouse. It is fascinating how specific aromas, from freshly cut grass to baby shampoo, can immediately transport our minds to places where our memories have a strong association with that particular smell. It is one of our most powerful senses.

The age-old adage 'Stop and smell the roses' is a perfect illustration of the connection between our senses and our awareness of being in the present moment. Whatever is happening in your day, pausing for just a few seconds to breathe in the scent of a flower will immediately bring you back to your senses, and back into your body and mind, in the here and now.

AROMATIC
HERBS

Find a fresh herb, such as parsley, mint, rosemary or coriander, and pick a sprig, scrunching up the leaves with your fingers.

Close your eyes and hold the herb close to your nose so that you can inhale deeply and smell the oils released by the crushed leaves.

What are the characteristics of the scent? Is it fresh or musky, delicate or strong? Does it bring any memories with it? What are those memories – are they fleeting images, vague feelings, or detailed scenes?

Focus on your breath and the aroma entering your body. Is there an emotion associated with the scent? How does it make you feel?

TOUCH

As humans, we find touch deeply nourishing and balancing, and yet in our modern lives, we might go through the entire day without engaging very much with this sense. We tend to touch or hold things without thinking about them much.

Think about the phrase 'to be in touch', meaning to be connected with oneself, with one's environment or with others.

Keep a lookout for interesting textures or materials. Even as you open a door, connect with the moment that you take hold of the handle and sense the weight of the door. When you pick up paper from the photocopier or printer, take a moment to notice and enjoy the warmth that lingers on the pages. If you are wearing something that is made from a soft or pleasant fabric, allow yourself to run your fingers over it, enjoying the sensation. If you're outside, perhaps you might take off your shoes and explore how it feels to walk barefoot on the cool grass, or take the time to notice the sensations on your skin as the breeze plays over your body, or a sudden burst of warmth as the sun emerges from behind a cloud. Think about how many of these feelings we miss every day, just because we are not aware enough to notice them.

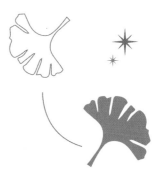

FOCUS ON FEELING

To practise becoming more aware of your sense of touch, choose an interesting object near you that calls out to be felt.

Perhaps it has a pleasing or ergonomic shape, like a paperweight or a soft toy. Perhaps it's spiky or uncomfortable to hold.

Take it in your hands, close your eyes, and explore the object purely through the way it feels to touch it. Is it cool or warm, rough or smooth? Where are its imperfections, those tiny things that make it unique? Does it feel the same as it looks? Is there anything about it that interests or surprises you?

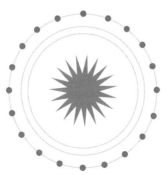

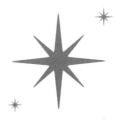

In today's busy world, there is no shortage of sound – in fact, we often end up trying to block it out with earplugs or headphones. Too much sound can, of course, be overwhelming. But when you allow yourself to absorb the background sounds around you, you may find there are fascinating details that heighten your sense of presence and give you a feeling of understanding of where you are in the world. Sound is, after all, vibration, and so your body constantly resonates with the sounds around you. If you can pay attention to the sensation of listening with your whole body, you become truly aware.

Absorb the background sounds around you, you may find there are fascinating details that heighten your sense of presence.

Today, spend a few minutes just listening to and absorbing the sounds around you: the distant hum of traffic, the trickling of the radiator, the faraway drone of a plane overhead, the tapping of your colleague typing, the faint ringing of a phone on the other side of the office, the muffled sound of a TV or radio in the next room. Bathe in it, absorb it, and experience it mindfully.

SOUND BATHING

There is a wonderful practice that is growing in popularity called 'sound bathing'. Singing bowls and other sound vessels are used as a means of meditation in which sounds are absorbed by the body and mind. This can be a powerful and deeply soothing experience. Look online and see if there are any sound bath classes or workshops near you.

Alternatively, you can search for a sound bath on YouTube and try it out at home. Use headphones for a more immersive experience.

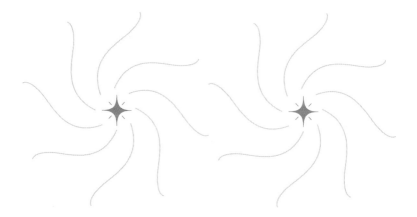

TASTE

We already discussed eating mindfully on page 38, but connecting with taste is a great way to feel present and mindful in the moment, and there are so many ways to do it. Perhaps you've just brushed your teeth; how does the minty aftertaste of the toothpaste feel on your tongue? Next time you sip your drink, linger in the moment and think about the taste. Is it bitter, sweet, savoury, refreshing? As you did with smell, consider whether the taste brings back any memories or summons up a particular feeling. Focus on that and explore it as you eat.

BEING IN YOUR BODY

When we talk about our bodies, we often use language that distances us from them. We say, 'I have a body', not 'I am a body'. Sometimes, we are cruel to our bodies. We criticize them and resent them for not being the

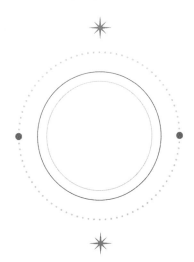

shape we think they should be, or for not being as strong or as tall or as healthy or as young as we want them to be.

But the human body is a miraculous thing. As you sit here reading this, millions of cells are working hard to keep you alive and functioning. Your heart is beating, your lungs are breathing, your muscles are working to hold you in whatever position you're currently in. Your digestive system is breaking down the last thing you ate; your brain is thinking about the words on the page, but it's also managing hundreds of other functions, many of which you're not even aware of.

Perhaps we should treasure these magical bodies of ours a little more. Over the coming pages, we'll be looking at ways to more mindfully and consciously inhabit your body, becoming present within it.

Connecting with taste is a great way to feel present and mindful in the moment.

✳

Next time you sip your drink, linger in the moment and think about the taste.

✳

QUICK BODY SCAN

We will explore a more in-depth body scan on page 66, but this mindful exercise is a useful tool to employ if you don't have much time, but just need to reconnect with your body and your presence.

You will need a chair and a quiet space where you won't be distracted by other people coming into the space. Noises beyond the space are natural and are part of the exercise.

Read through the exercise in full and then try it, as it's best to do it with your eyes closed.

1. Sit with your back comfortably straight against the chair and with your feet flat on the floor.

2. Close your eyes and breathe normally, bringing your attention to your breath.

3. Gradually, bring your attention to the crown of your head and just sense if there is a 'presence' there. Try not to 'look' with your mind, but feel this part of your body and whether there is any energy or sensation there.

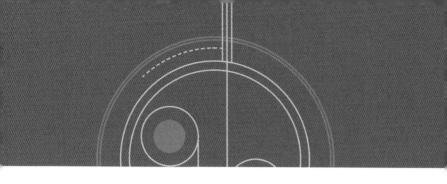

4. Now scan each part of your body, moving down from your head towards your toes, again simply bringing an awareness rather than 'looking'. How does your right hand feel versus your left? Can you detect a slightly different level of presence?

5. Are there any areas where you can't really detect any presence? Notice these areas; there is no need to try and change anything or do anything.

6. When you have scanned your whole body, gently bring your focus back to the breath, bring your awareness into the room in which you are sitting, and when you are ready, open your eyes.

Try to take this feeling of being present in your body with your as you continue with your day.

COMFORTABLE IN YOUR OWN SKIN

Journal prompt: When are you comfortable in your own skin?

'Wherever my travels may lead, paradise is where I am.'
– Voltaire

Think about a typical situation in your life when you feel comfortable and content; when you feel good in yourself, at ease and relaxed. Perhaps it's when you are outside in nature, or curled up on the sofa with a book. Perhaps it's when you're sitting in a cosy café and chatting with friends; perhaps it's when you're out jogging or riding your bike, feeling the wind in your hair and the energy coursing through your limbs as you move.

Try to think of several examples, then take a few minutes to journal about them. Pay attention to how these situations make you feel, physically and emotionally.

Having an awareness of what sorts of situation make you feel comfortable and content is a valuable resource, and

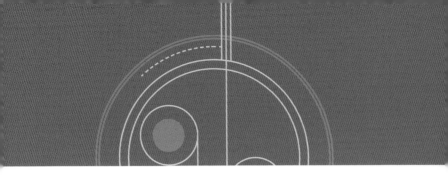

it can be very empowering – whenever you feel as if your emotional resources are getting low, you can seek out these situations and draw on them to help you recharge. Taking the time to journal about them can help increase your awareness of why these situations are so restorative to you, and may help you identify other situations that will have a similarly soothing impact.

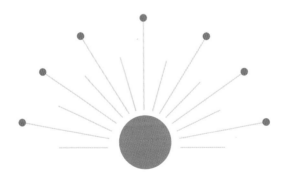

MINDFUL MOVEMENT

It is easy to spend too much time in our own heads, amid a whirl of circulating ideas, plans and constant commentary, and we often lose access to much of the rest of the body.

We need to practise mindful movement as a vehicle for insight and understanding about ourselves. The following exercises will help you explore mindful movement and feel a sense of presence in your body and in the moment.

1. Sit with your back straight and your hands resting on your thighs.

2. Very slowly, lift your dominant hand and, moment by moment, experience moving it through the air.

3. Practise slowly and mindfully reaching out to any small object in front of you. Pick it up slowly and feel the sensation of holding it. Then, stretch out your arm again and return the object to where it came from.

4. Keep practising this for several minutes to make the connection between mindfulness and the movement of your hand.

YOGA FLOW

The mindful movements practised in yoga can help us carve out a space of quiet and connection in the busy world in which we live. Any kind of yoga can make a valuable part of your mindfulness practice, so it's worth looking into local classes or even finding a tutorial online. For now, though, try the following simple movements, giving two or three minutes to each. Always remember to do them with relaxed and mindful breathing.

1. Stand with your feet close together. Roll your neck first in one direction and then in the other.

2. Raise your shoulders up to your ears, and then relax while lowering your shoulders. Squeeze your shoulder blades together, then relax.

3. Raise your arms above your head and hook your thumbs together, breathing in and out from your stomach.

4. Allow both arms to hang down, fingers pointing to your toes. Now gently stretch your back, without forcing it.

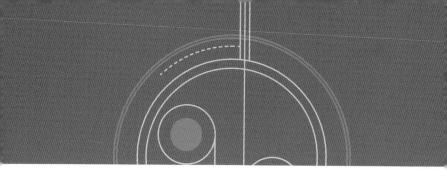

5. Lift your arms straight above your head, and point your fingers towards the ceiling. Slowly lean your body to the left, feeling a stretch on your right side. Repeat, leaning your body to the right, feeling a stretch on your left side.

6. Lie on your back with your feet close together. Lift both feet off the ground, hold for a few seconds and release.

7. Lie on your back and bend your knees. Place your arms around your shins, then lift your knees and head, drawing them close to each other.

8. Stand up straight and extend your arms straight out ahead of you. Bend your knees.

9. Very slowly, moment by moment, raise your arms until your fingertips point to the sky. Then, keeping your arms straight, lower them down, bending your back slowly until your fingertips point towards your toes. Allow your torso to hang down for several seconds without forcing your back to bend further. Then straighten your back and come back to standing, letting your arms hang down at the sides of your body, with your chest expanding.

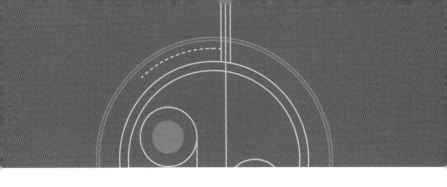

10. Breathe mindfully.

11. Take a rest. Lie down with your arms at your sides and your feet just a couple of inches apart. Be still. Breathe gently. Rest for at least five to ten minutes.

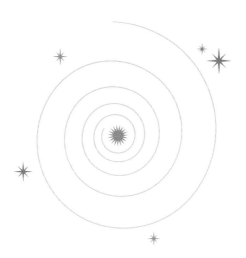

HANDS

We use our hands in almost every moment of our lives, whether we're eating, typing, holding something, drawing or touching a loved one – but how often do we really notice them?

Practising mindfulness of the hands can reveal much about the self. In a way, the hands are an extension of our inner life. What happens to the hands in a given moment reveals much about our state of mind. When we feel nervous or unsettled, the vibrations of this state are often revealed through the fingers tapping on the knee, or by the repeated clasping and unclasping of the fist. Mind and body are so intimately connected that our hand movements often serve as a public advertisement for what is taking place in our minds.

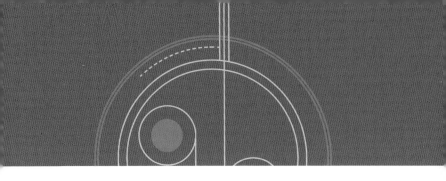

1. Put this book down and place your hands in your lap. Rest one hand of top of the other with the tips of your thumbs touching each other.

2. Make sure that your back is straight and that you are sitting comfortably. Relax into this position, breathing in and out deeply.

3. Hold this position for five minutes, keeping your body as calm as possible.

4. Direct your mindfulness to the sensations in your hands. Notice whether they are tense or relaxed, warm or cool, dry or moist.

5. Slowly raise one hand, with your fingers outstretched, to the level of the shoulder, and then slowly return the hand to the lap. Repeat this methodical movement with the other hand.

6. Practise this technique daily, and appreciate the calmness and freedom that mindfulness of the hands gives you from the unnecessary demands you place on yourself and the world.

FEELING YOUR FEET

To live mindfully, we need to bring full attention to the way we use our feet. We often think that our home is where we live, or where our heart is. In spiritual practice, our home is where our feet are. Where are your feet right now? Do you have both feet firmly on the ground, or is one foot on the floor and the other crossed over your leg, hanging in the air? If it is, adjust your position so that both feet are on the floor. Now stop and notice the contact of your feet with the floor.

What does that feel like?

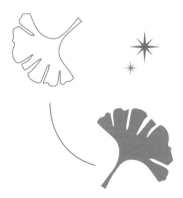

Harmonizing body and mind gives us a sense of inner peace throughout our whole being. We feel at ease, comfortable and stable within our immediate environment. There is spaciousness in our outlook and a fullness to our lives, whether active or not. When we feel this harmony of body and mind, we place demands neither on the world nor on ourselves. We experience a natural equilibrium and a balanced relationship with every one of our senses.

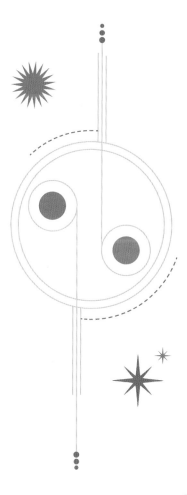

FULL BODY SCAN

The following meditation practice points to a direct relationship between mind and body. It is a practice that can be done daily, and is particularly beneficial for those who need to develop a harmonious relationship rather than an adversarial one between body and mind. Place your attention directly on your body, starting with your head and going down to your feet. Attune your mindfulness to the immediate experience of the body sensations themselves. This is a subtle moment-to-moment practice, in which every single part of the body is experienced.

1. Lie down or sit comfortably on a chair with your back straight. Start by focusing your attention on the top of your head, then slowly move down your neck, shoulders and arms.

2. Next, move your attention slowly down your back to your buttocks, and down your front to your genitals.

3. Finally, move your focus slowly from the top of each leg down to your toes.

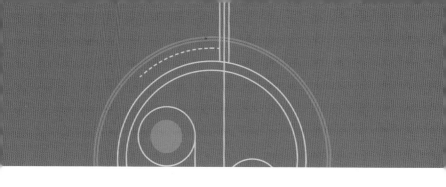

4. This scanning of your body may take anywhere from five to thirty minutes. When you're ready, reverse the process, starting from your feet and working slowly up to the top of your head.

5. As you gradually move your attention down and then up your body, experience all the sensations – vibrations, aches, pain, tingling, throbbing, itching, warmth, coolness, numbness – the whole range of pleasant and unpleasant feelings. Don't try to resist the feelings, or favour some over others. Just notice them.

6. On completion of this practice, allow your body to be completely still. Be fully present to the presence of your whole body.

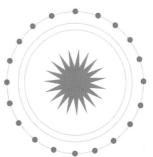

PERCEIVING PAIN IN A BODY SCAN

Some people experience pain in certain locations in the body, and this can be particularly noticeable during body-scanning meditations.

If this is true for you, it can be useful to spend more time in that area of pain, quietly but firmly turning your attention to the pain. Explore it from the outer edges to the very centre, so the mindfulness penetrates deeper and deeper into the pain. Is the pain very specific, or does it have blurred outer edges that are difficult to define?

Can you give the pain a colour?

Spend more time in that area of pain, quietly but firmly turning your attention to the pain.

Now slowly move on to the next area, taking notice of and appreciating all the locations where there isn't pain.

As you do this, try to imagine yourself as a watcher or observer, so that you can acknowledge the pain without being consumed by it.

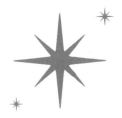

FOCUS ON FEELING

Because the mind and body are intrinsically linked, emotional pain, as well as physical pain, can manifest in the body. The following practical exercise will help dissolve contractions around painful feelings and thoughts, bringing harmony and alignment to body and mind. This is an invaluable practice.

1. Sit comfortably in a chair with a straight back. Adopt a relaxed posture. Close your eyes and turn your attention inwards to see if there is a particular place in your body where you experience an unpleasant feeling. It could be in your chest, stomach or another part of your body. Notice the outer edges of that feeling; notice the centre of it. Stay quietly focused and in touch with its location in your body.

2. What is that feeling telling you? How would you describe it? Experience the feeling in your body. Try to find one or two words for the feeling.

3. As you examine the feeling, consider this: what do you need to understand here? What insight is needed to resolve the issue that is causing this feeling?

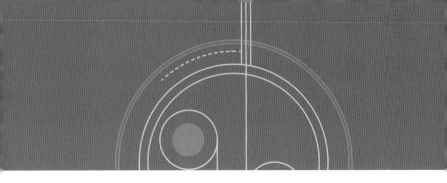

Various thoughts and conclusions may arise in answer to these questions. A genuine insight or moment of clarity will produce some kind of qualitative shift in the feeling, which may be temporary or long-standing.

Let any understanding that emerges rest within you. Avoid indulging in unpleasant feelings or emotions. Bear in mind what you see clearly.

The understanding may show itself simply and directly. The feeling may signify acceptance, change, avoidance, patience. The feeling may be asking you to do something: to let go of something, to make contact with someone, to breathe more mindfully, to dance. If you feel unsure or confused, turn your attention back to the bare feeling, noticing again which part of your body experiences the feeling. Explore that region of your body again. Let it tell you what it needs to.

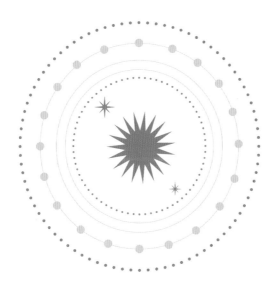

WHERE DO YOU FEEL STRONG?

It is a human tendency to focus on where we wish to improve, often ignoring the positive aspects of ourselves. Imagine a tree, hundreds of years old, with an amazing root system and a strong, yet flexible trunk, with limbs that sway in the wind without breaking.

Where is the energy in your body and in your sense of self, right now? Is the flame burning strongly, or do you need to tend the fire and give attention to any of these places or aspects of yourself?

Where is your greatest potential that lies within?

YOUR FAVOURITE TIME OF DAY

Some of us are morning people; others are night owls. Some of us find that we get a burst of energy in the afternoons, while others enjoy the sense of calm, reflection and winding down that comes with early evening. Take some time to think about the time of day that you most appreciate. What is it about this time of day that stands out? What feelings are associated with it? Is it a time full of potential, or perhaps a time filled with peace or the joy of being with others?

Each day, the sun rises and sets, reminding us that nothing is permanent, that time can never stand still. But by focusing our awareness, we bring richness, detail and colour to the experience of every day, from the moment we awake to the moment we drift off to sleep.

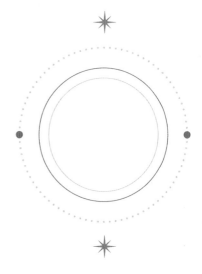

TREASURING THE EVERYDAY

Think about a simple activity or moment that occurs every day, but gives you a sense of warmth or comfort. It might be the relaxing feeling of walking through your front door at the end of a long day at work, or the pleasure of walking past that lovely garden on your way to the bus stop. It could be as small as the feeling of splashing your face with water in the morning, or the pleasing ritual of making a cup of herbal tea before bed. These seemingly small things really do have an impact, especially when we bring our awareness to them.

Journal about your chosen activity or moment in loving detail, trying to capture every aspect of the experience and why you treasure it. Drawing your attention to it in this way will help you notice and appreciate it even more.

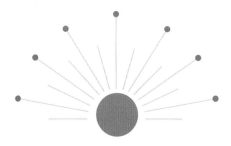

CLARITY

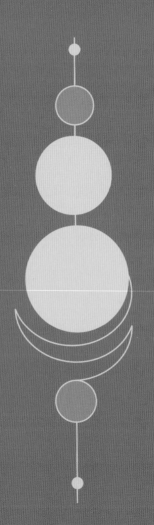

Let distractions fall away and allow yourself to see things as they are.

'How've you been?'

'Oh, good. You know. Busy. Busy, busy, busy.'

Sound familiar?

So many of us work far too many hours, sitting at our desks or glued to our emails from dawn until late at night. It's not just that we can't find time to relax – we don't know how to. We've lost the ability to slow down, to stop. Even when we're not physically at work, our minds are busy, running through to-do lists, obligations, worries.

An unsettled mind blocks our ability to see things as they are. We get caught up in our imaginations and sacrifice peace of mind to our worries and expectations. We might get tied up in imagining different scenarios or making assumptions about how other people are feeling. All of this can cloud our judgement and leave us feeling overwhelmed and uncertain.

In order to see things clearly, we need to learn to cultivate a quiet, calm and still mind on a daily basis, allowing ourselves to settle into the present moment, and see it for what it really is. With this comes clarity, and a sense of space and freedom.

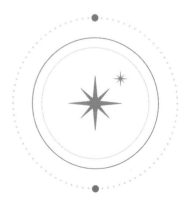

BE STILL

If you habitually feel tired or stressed out, pay attention to the energy you waste through scratching, fidgeting, changing position, crossing and uncrossing your legs or fiddling around with a pen or paper clip, an item of clothing or a strand of hair. Even when we think we're sitting still, we're often still moving in some small way, or holding ourselves tense. Think about it now. How are you sitting or standing as you read this? Perhaps your jaw is clenched, or your shoulders are hunched.

To live a mindful life, consider the different ways in which you expend energy through excess movement and restlessness. Practise being calm and still instead. Sit in a meditative pose and you will find

that you can conserve the energy of the mind and body so that it can be used for purposes that are more important.

The practical benefits of mindfulness include understanding how to conserve energy, and not dissipating it through restless movement. If you work and work, your body will eventually give up in protest. Genuine mindfulness will help to reveal to us such unhealthy patterns and give us the power to make changes and seek out peace and rest before we burn out.

Try to find times throughout the day to sit in stillness and position yourself firmly in the present moment.

At the heart of any mindful practice is awareness – the art of paying attention.

TAKING NOTICE

With so many distractions in our modern lives and in our minds, it is not always easy to access a state of awareness. Have you ever got to work and realized you can't really remember a moment of your commute? You might spend much of the day on autopilot, catching the same train, buying the same type of coffee from the same shop, so that when you take even a few minutes to focus yourself consciously on your state of awareness – even if that means simply noticing how unaware you have been – you might be surprised by the richness of that experience. Try it now:

1. Take a few moments to settle into yourself and your immediate environment.

2. Take a few deep, easy breaths and try to get in touch with a sense of awareness, a sense of your presence and the energy within and around you.

You might simply notice the thoughts running around your mind (which, in itself, lessens their intensity), or you might stop to notice the details in your surroundings – what you can hear, smell and see.

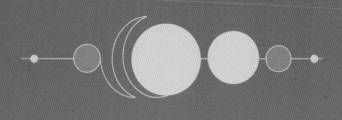

3. In your mind (or out loud, if you prefer), say, 'Right now, in this moment, I am aware that...' – and allow yourself to explore the moment you are in.

You can do this anywhere, at any time of day, making it an ideal exercise for grounding yourself and re-rooting yourself with a sense of clarity and calm in the present moment.

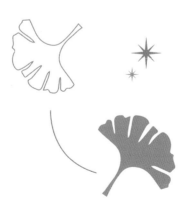

WHEN THINGS GO WRONG

Mindfulness and the clarity it brings can be extremely valuable tools to tap in to when things go wrong. Our brains are busy places, and as a species we are prone to analysing situations and trying to work out what might happen. Sometimes, of course, this is necessary, and it keeps us safe – for example, when we judge potential risks before making a manoeuvre when driving. However, there are times when we get lost in these what-ifs and worries, and it can be hard to separate them from what is actually happening

When things go wrong – if we make a mistake at work, disagree with a friend or don't pass a test – we can become overwhelmed as our minds go into overdrive and we catastrophise. That mistake at work

When things go wrong we can become overwhelmed as our minds go into overdrive.

takes on gigantic proportions; we might begin to doubt our ability, or worry that our job is at risk. We might replay the conversation we had with our friend, analysing every sentence, wondering if they misunderstood us, or we them, and if they are now thinking badly of us. If we fail a test, we might begin to feel as though that failure is insurmountable, and extends to every other area of our lives.

In situations like this, practising mindfulness can help us to differentiate between what we're worried about happening, and what actually is happening. Rather than allowing ourselves to react as if we're in the midst of a crisis, we can turn an inconvenience or a challenge into an opportunity to develop calmness, contentment and patience. We can learn from mistakes at work, we can work on improving our communication with our friends, we can calmly consider where the test went wrong and take steps to improve for next time.

Seeing things as they actually are can help us stay calm and purposeful, even when things are hard.

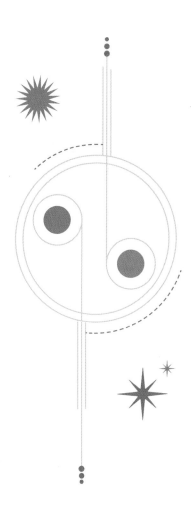

WALL OF SCREENS MEDITATION

When we're juggling lots of conflicting demands, it can feel like we're being pulled in all directions – you need to finish that report before the deadline, you need to remember to pick up milk on the way home, you need to call the plumber, you need to pay that bill, you promised your partner you'd book those tickets, you have an alarming number of unread 'urgent' emails, and you're pretty sure there's something else, too, although you can't quite remember what it is...

There are days when it can feel like the whole word is barking orders at us, and we're stretched too thin and completely overwhelmed.

This meditation uses vizualisation to help you try and block out some of the noise and distractions so that you can move through your day with a little more ease.

Find somewhere quiet to sit for a few minutes. Read the meditation through before you start, because it's best to do this with your eyes closed.

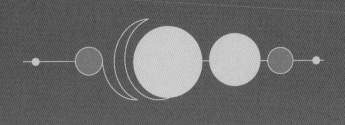

1. Sit comfortably, with your back straight and your feet firmly planted on the floor. Take a few deep breaths.

2. Now – and this is going to sound counterintuitive – let the noise in. Imagine you're sitting in front of a wall of TV screens, and each screen is showing a different channel. One screen has your boss, asking you when you're going to finish the report. One shows the supermarket, all the things you're supposed to be picking up. On every screen is a face or an image representing the many, many things that are fighting for your attention. And they're all talking at you at once.

3. Imagine you're holding a remote control. Slowly and deliberately, lift up the remote control and point it at one of the screens.

4. Press the 'off' button and imagine the screen going blank.

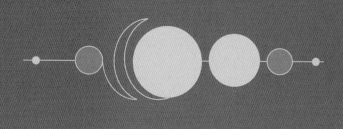

5. Keep doing this, working your way from screen to screen, until all the screens are blank and the room is quiet. Sit in the calm clarity of this moment and allow it to wash over you.

6. When you're ready, open your eyes.

Of course, we can't actually just switch off our demands and obligations, but this exercise is a great way of helping you calm down when it all gets overwhelming. And once you're calmer, you can begin to see clearly which things to prioritise, and come up with a plan of action.

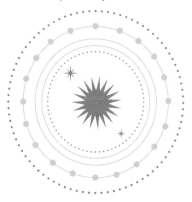

INTUITION

Just as we explored the physical senses on pages 46–52, mindfulness can help you develop an awareness of what some people might call your 'sixth sense': intuition.

As your sense of clarity and awareness of the present moment grows, along with your awareness of your sense of self and others, you may find you become more in tune with a sort of inner knowing: your intuition, your gut instinct, your inner wisdom.

Can you think of a time when you paid attention to this 'sixth sense' and it help you out, or helped others? Or even a time when you dismissed it and regretted that choice later on? Perhaps you had a sense that you should or shouldn't go to a certain event, and following

that sense led to an important experience. Perhaps you felt an urge to reach out to someone you hadn't spoken to for a while, only to find that they were feeling lost and in need of support. Perhaps you received two job offers and just knew, deep inside, that one was better for you, even if the other paid more. Spend some time reflecting on that experience of intuition or instinct. Understanding how it felt can help you to identify it in future.

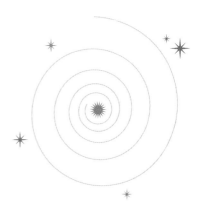

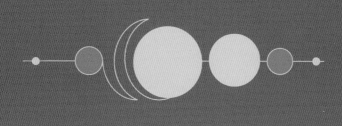

Journal prompt: What does your heart say?

We live in a society that tends to value intellectual intelligence over emotional intelligence. Because of this, it isn't always very easy to listen deeply to what your heart is saying. There is where journaling can be incredibly helpful, especially when you allow yourself to write in a stream-of-consciousness fashion, not worrying about forming specific sentences or thinking about where your writing might go.

Take a moment to settle and sit quietly, breathing naturally.

Imagine breathing into your heart space. Do this for a few deep, gentle breaths. Breathe in through the nose and out through the mouth, letting go of any tension with your out-breath.

What does your heart say?

When you're ready, pick up your pen and simply write. It doesn't matter if you start a sentence without knowing how it will end. Let your heart tell you.

DEER IN THE
FOREST MEDITATION

Read through this meditation in full before you begin, as it's best to do it with your eyes closed. Alternatively, you can record yourself reading this page aloud and then listen to the recording as you meditate.

Find a comfortable place to sit and gently bring your attention to your breath, allowing your thoughts to begin to slow down and settle. Become the observer of your thoughts as they drift in and out of your mind, like clouds across the sky.

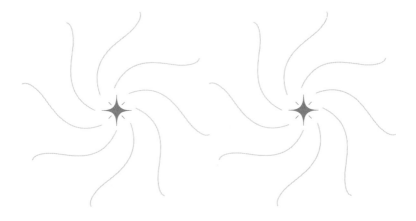

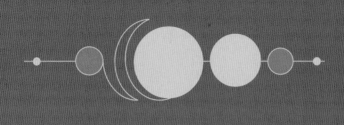

1. Now, imagine that you are walking through a forest, with sunlight filtering through the leaves of the trees, the smell of the earth beneath your feet, and the sounds of nature all around you. You are walking at a natural pace, noticing the details: the patterns of the bark, the signs of the season, the cool breeze on your skin.

2. Ahead of you on the path, you see a beautiful doe. The doe has spotted you at the same time and is looking towards you with calm curiosity. You stand completely still, relaxed but motionless, looking straight into the eyes of the doe, which are full of nature's wisdom.

3. Is there a question you wish to ask the doe? What question is rising up in your mind? Go ahead and ask.

4. Now look deeply into the doe's eyes. Relax and wait for the answer.

MONO NO AWARE

'Mono no aware' is a phrase linked to the Japanese aesthetics of impermanence, the melancholic beauty that is found in the fact that nothing in life is permanent. The concept of impermanence is often linked to nature, where the seasons show us so poignantly and beautifully that nothing remains the same.

This concept is often symbolized by the cherry blossoms that bloom in Japan each spring, staying for such a short time. They are stunningly beautiful – perhaps even more so due to the fact that their time is so fleeting.

Explore the idea of impermanence in your own life. Can you detect its beauty, even its sadness? Perhaps you can see it in the way your child is growing up, getting older, making you want to treasure these moments when they're still little? Perhaps you see it in a beautiful

'Yesterday I was so clever, so I wanted to change the world. Today, I am wise, so I am changing myself.'

Rumi

bouquet of flowers that are filling the room with colour and scent, but will eventually fade and wilt? It can be found in the simplest of things: tea doesn't stay hot, ice cream melts, trees drop their leaves.

Developing a sense of the way impermanence and change flow through our lives can help us develop clarity around what truly matters to us in each moment, helping us to become more thoughtful and appreciative of the gifts that are all around us.

EVIDENCE TO
THE CONTRARY

It's easy to become very attached to a fixed sense of identity, when in reality we can change at any given moment, if we are willing to let go. If you feel you aren't a very courageous, creative or generous person, the truth is that you can be any of those things – and you have been all of those things, at various moments of your life.

Today is the day to stop building up the piles of evidence that support any fixed or limiting ideas you have about yourself or others. Today, look for evidence to the contrary.

Developing a sense of the way impermanence and change flow through our lives can help us develop clarity around what truly matters to us.

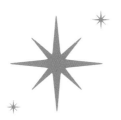

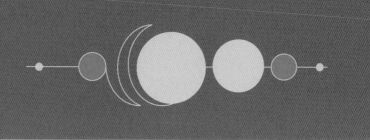

Journal prompt: What is blocking you?

As we work on developing a sense of clarity and awareness, we become better able to identify those areas in our life where things are not quite as we want them to be. Use this journaling exercise to dig a little deeper and gain some insight into what these areas are for you.

Is there a place in your life where you feel there is a sticking point, or a block of some kind, between where you are right now and where you wish to be?

Sit with this question for a few minutes and try to identify an answer or answers. Try not to censor the answers that come, but accept them as they are, and write them down.

Once you have identified these blocks, begin to explore whether you have positioned them as external forces that you feel are beyond your control, such as another person or a rule or convention.

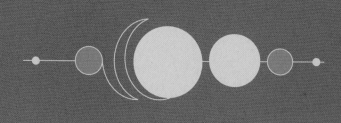

Now imagine the same block or obstacle, but bring it within yourself. You are no longer powerless. Imagine how you might go around the obstacle or release its power over you, even for these few minutes. What choices would you need to make? Spend some time writing about this.

Often, blocks are of our own making, and when we give ourselves time and space to consider them, we might be able to identify this. Old habits and patterns have incredible strength over our behaviours and thoughts; they are a well-worn groove. Is there an old limiting belief you have about yourself that might be contributing to your block? What if you questioned that belief?

This journaling exercise can help us identify areas in our lives where we are being held back by limiting beliefs rather than genuine limitations. With the clarity this brings, we can take steps towards focusing on what matters most.

SHINE ONE CORNER

It is easy to get tangled up in worrying about all the things in the world that we wish were different, and often we get caught on those things over which we have no control or influence. Although it's admirable to want to make a difference and solve big problems, that's not possible for all of us – or most of us. You may not be able to fix everything, but you can 'shine one corner', as Suzuki says. The small, tangible things over which we do have control can ultimately have a significant impact on us and those around us. You may not be able to solve the economic crisis, but you can take your elderly neighbour's bins out for them. You might not be able to prevent a friend's marriage from crumbling, but you can cook them dinner and offer them nourishment and care. You may not be able to buy your dream home, but you can make your bed, wash your dishes and make the home you do inhabit, your own little corner of the world, a space that is pleasant to be in.

How can you shine one corner?

'We say, to shine one corner of the world – just one corner. If you shine one corner, then people around you will feel better.'

Shunryu Suzuki

WHAT DO YOU WANT TO DO TODAY

Often, we can find ourselves so tied up in all the things we think we should be doing, that it can be easy to lose sight of why we are doing them – or whether we really want to. Sometimes, we do things in order to have done them rather than actively experiencing them in the moment, such as going to the gym with a sense of obligation and a feeling of ticking something off a list, rather than seeing it as an opportunity to connect with our bodies and engage in purposeful movement.

Instead of your usual to-do list, this exercise is about engaging with what you want to do and why. With the sense of clarity it brings, you may find that tasks that felt like chores or obligations become more appealing when viewed through a more mindful and deliberate lens.

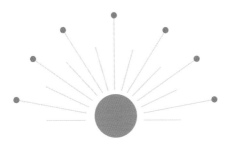

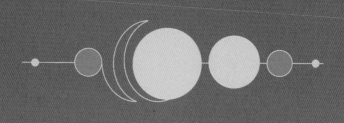

Think about the word 'yes'. Feel it. Think about where it lands in your body. What colour is it? What shape? When you say or hear the word 'yes', what are the thoughts and feelings that arise? Is there anything you really wish you could say 'yes' to?

Just as we need to listen to the whispers of our hearts when it comes to saying 'yes', the same is true when it comes to saying 'no'.

Consider the word 'no'. How does it feel? Is it heavy, difficult to hold? What does it bring up for you? Do you feel uncomfortable saying 'no' to other people? Or do you tell yourself 'no' too often, out of fear and anxiety?

And – and this is a big one – what would it be like to say 'no' to something you didn't want to do? What about if you said 'yes' to something you want, when you've been telling yourself 'no'? How would that feel? What would happen?

There is immense power in these two tiny words.

FOCUS WHEEL

With this sense of clarity and understanding around 'yes' and 'no', try writing a to-do list. This isn't a traditional list of tasks for the day. The purpose here is to consider how you will align your daily actions with your bigger goals or values – your 'yeses' and your 'nos'.

In other words, it is a to-do list written in awareness.

If you like, you can consider items that might usually be included on your typical to-do list, but try to view them from this more mindful angle – not because you feel you 'should' do them, but because of how they align with your purpose or values. For example, you might decide to include going to the supermarket on your list, not because you 'should' go, but because you intend to buy food that will support and strengthen your body and be a way of caring for yourself.

If you could only do one thing today, what would it be?

What will you say 'no' to today?

What will you say 'yes' to?

CONNECTION

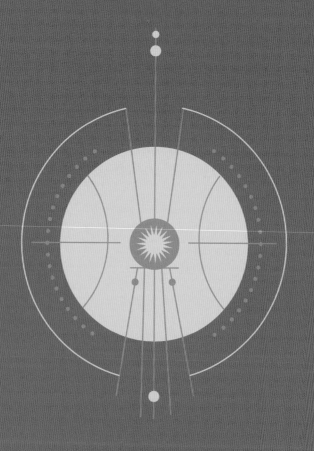

Connect consciously and with your full attention.

We use the word 'connection' a lot these days, but most of the time, we're talking about the internet! Thanks to the wonders of modern technology, these days we are more 'connected' than ever – we can speak to people on the other side of the world, and access news and information at the click of a button. There's nothing wrong with this – in fact, it's all pretty wonderful – but it's important not to mistake access and surface-level connection for real, in-depth, meaningful connection.

Mindfulness can help us to understand and appreciate connection on a deeper level, and develop a sense of how everything around us ties together, from the interactions and links we see in nature to the relationships we have with others.

When we feel connected, we feel grounded, focused, supported, understood and valued. When we feel disconnected, we feel cut adrift, alone and uncertain.

True connection is about mindful, active listening, awareness and appreciation. It can improve our relationships and bring meaning to our lives.

Mindfulness can help us to understand and appreciate connection on a deeper level.

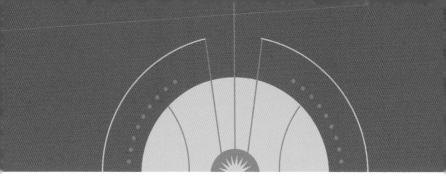

Journal prompt: What touches your soul?

This journal prompt can help you explore the idea of connection by identifying the things that make you feel connected; the moments or experiences that resonate with you and help you feel like part of something bigger than you.

Where is the sense of magic in your life? What helps you come into awareness of your own self, awareness of others and awareness of your environment?

If we are to connect with ourselves and how we feel, so that we may then fully connect with those around us, it is a good idea to notice those things that seem to help us feel aware.

It might be those moments when the natural world takes your breath away, or when you stop to catch the scent of a flower. Perhaps it is the kindness of a stranger, or the sound of a busker singing in the street, or reading the opening line of a favourite novel or poem.

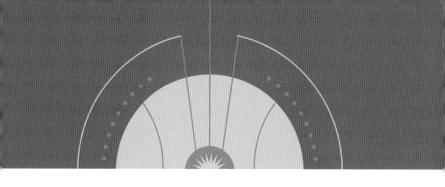

In your journal, describe some of these moments and think about what it is about them that sparks a sense of connection within you. What is it that you are feeling connected to? Is it another person, a sense of culture or history, or perhaps even the universe itself? Taking the time to examine these moments and hold them up to the light can help us appreciate them and experience them still more deeply.

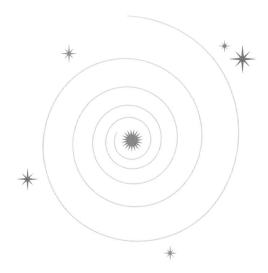

BREATHING WITH THE WORLD

As we breathe, the ongoing rhythm of inhalation and exhalation gives us the nourishment we need to live and eliminates the waste that would suffocate us if we could not let it go.

With every in-breath, we draw in oxygen, which the heart pumps through the lungs to fuel the life process in the cells of the body. With every out-breath, the cells' waste is pumped out in the form of carbon dioxide and released back into the air.

By contrast, the plants and trees around us absorb this carbon dioxide and create oxygen.

This cycle of mutual nourishment and elimination goes on throughout our lives, whether or not we are mindful of it.

Just thinking about it for a moment. There is something quite extraordinary about this whole process of organic life interacting moment by moment with the environment, connecting each of us with the world around us with every breath.

It's important not to mistake access and surface-level connection for real, in-depth, meaningful connection.

TREE
MEDITATION

This meditation can help you feel a sense of connection to the earth and the world around you. It's particularly useful for those days when you feel swept up in the blur and busy-ness of everyday life.

1. Picture a large tree, standing strong in the earth, its branches reaching upwards and outwards, extending towards the sky. Follow each branch with your mind's eye, from the trunk to the very tip of the smallest leaf.

2. Now consider the tree's roots. Although we can't see them, they are there, reaching outwards and downwards just as the branches reach, a vast network of connected tendrils that keep the tree nourished and hold it steady in the earth. Remember that every tree has the systems of branches that we can see, and the system of roots that we can't.

3. Consider the roots that hold you in place, and connect you to the earth. They are not physical in the way that the tree's roots are physical, but they tether and connect you in the same way. Your roots might be your family, your cultural history, your personal beliefs, your passions. They are the

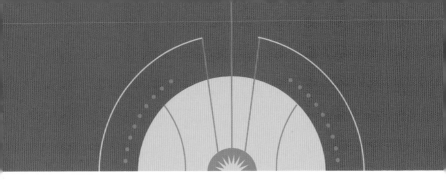

things that nourish you and connect you to the world. Like the tree's roots, they might be hidden, but they are powerful, and they are just as important to your wellbeing as the visible parts of your life.

4. As you breathe, imagine your own roots reaching deep into the earth, grounding you and keeping you connected to the things that matter most to you, even as you reach upwards towards your potential.

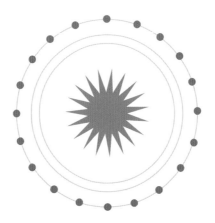

CONNECTING TO NATURE

Paying attention to the natural world is a powerful way to feel more connected. When you give your attention to nature, it will repay you a thousand times over with details full of wonder. The sheer amount of life that can be sensed in nature at any given moment is one of the most visceral reminders of presence there is. From the wildest of woods to the smallest of gardens, nature abounds. Even a plant pot contains a whole world in its soil; insects and microbes and plant life, all existing together. Next time you're in a garden, look around at the plants and the trees and the grass. Look at the birds flying overhead, the butterflies or bees. Think about the worms and other insects moving around in the earth beneath your feet. Look at the spiders spinning webs in among the bushes; see the slugs and snails moving slowly across the ground, or the ants marching purposefully across the path. Even in the middle of a city, nature finds a way: plants push their way up through concrete; birds make their nests in gutters and on rooftops.

When we feel connected, we feel grounded.

Nature stimulates all our senses and reminds us of where we are. Taking the time to mindfully observe and connect with the natural world, whether you take a walk in the woods, sit in your garden, or spend your lunchbreak in a city park, can bring a sense of calm and serenity to your day.

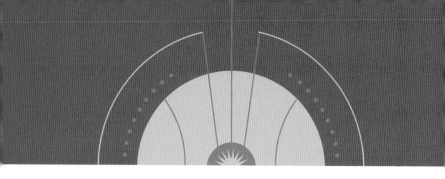

Journal prompt: The weather

It's common – and natural – to find ourselves indulging in a bit of a grumble about the weather. We might complain that it's too cold, or too rainy – but we also tend to moan when it's too hot, or when the weather has been so dry for so long that the grass is parched and scorched.

For this journal prompt, try describing your favourite kind of weather in as much detail as you can. How does it make you feel? What are the smells you associate with this weather? Why do you love it so much?

Now think about a type of weather you are less keen on. Try to focus the same kind of loving attention on this weather that you just gave to your favourite weather, and write about it. Perhaps, despite its faults, you love the freshly washed look everything has the morning after a rainy night.

Mindfulness can help us find joy in the ordinary and the mundane, and even the things we don't usually enjoy.

CLOUD GAZING

Staring up at the clouds and trying to find faces and patterns is something a lot of us did as children, but often we stop doing it as adults. We're usually too busy, and tend to look straight ahead or at the ground (or our phones!) as we walk.

Taking a moment to examine the clouds reminds us to stop staring at our feet and instead to look up at the sky. The patterns and shapes that clouds create are awe-inspiring, and connect us immediately with the world, the weather and the atmosphere. From wispy cirrus strands to big cotton-wool cumulus clumps, or heavy storm clouds that roll in without warning, clouds paint a picture above our heads every day.

And – like our thoughts – the clouds pass. They are impermanent, drifting across the sky and changing even as they travel.

Take some time to examine the clouds today. If you can, lie on the ground and gaze up at them like you did when you were a child. What can you see? How does it feel to watch them?

GRATITUDE FOR WHAT IS

Numerous studies have found that practising and developing gratitude can benefit both physical and mental health. Researchers at Northeastern University, Boston, MA, found that people who consciously felt a sense of gratitude each day became more patient and found it easier to make decisions. Other studies have discovered that feelings of gratitude are linked to healthy habits such as exercising and eating well. And it might sound obvious, but it's worth remembering that gratitude is beneficial to our relationships and the way we feel about life in general, boosting feelings of happiness and wellbeing.

Gratitude is beneficial to our relationships and the way we feel about life in general.

In short, mindfully practising gratitude can help us feel more connected and in sync with the world and the people around us, improving our quality of life and lifting our mood.

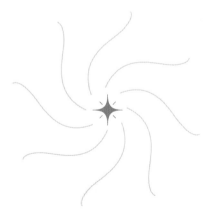

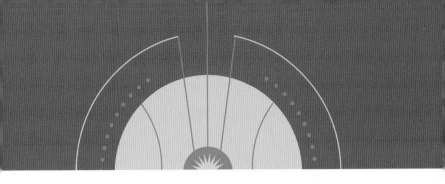

Journal prompt: Five minutes of gratitude

For this mindful writing exercise, which you can repeat at any time, all you have to do is let your mind and your heart run free, as you list everything you can think of in this moment for which you are grateful. You might be surprised by just how many things you can write down in five minutes.

There are no rules - absolutely anything or anyone can be included. You might think about big, abstract things, like your health, or love, or the coming of summer, or smaller, more definable (but no less important things), like the barista at your local coffee shop who always takes extra care with your order, or the person who smiled at you at the bus stop this morning.

Taking the time to consider these things, appreciate them and write them down can really highlight just how much there is in the world for which you feel grateful - and that can be a pretty wonderful feeling.

SHOWING GRATITUDE

✳

Showing our gratitude can be as simple and obvious as saying 'thank you', or it can be more subtle, expressed in an action or behaviour. Think about some of the things for which you are grateful – perhaps use the list you made on page 107. Consider these people and things, and think carefully about how you might show your gratitude in your own way. Perhaps you might wish to say thank you to the environment around you by consciously using less plastic, or you may wish to thank a loved one by calling them at the weekend, as they always love to chat.

Try to reframe actions that you know to be positive – like recycling, eating healthily, or cleaning your home – as acts of gratitude and appreciation. This will help you perform them with a sense of mindful connection and peace.

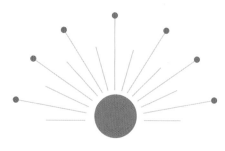

CONNECTION AND FRIENDSHIP

Our connections with other people are probably the most important connections we have.

Is it possible to live in a world without enemies, without hatred and without intolerance towards people we know and people we don't know? Is it possible to generate warmth and kindness towards everyone we meet?

Too often, we measure our friendships according to how others treat us, or how we treat them. The heart, free from these limitations, sees the falseness of this constant classifying of people or a particular person into different categories of approval and disapproval.

By going beyond such limitations, we move closer towards the ultimate truth. In deep friendship, expansive love and intimate connection, we know a life without limits or measurement. In the same way, the truth knows no limits.

Is it possible to live in a world without enemies?

Obviously, it is an enormous undertaking to break open the shell of armour around the heart to the degree that our friendship towards all existence pervades in all directions without compromise.

Genuine love can manifest itself in different expressions, such as friendship, kindness, gratitude, humility, appreciation, charity and compassion.

MEDITATE WITH A FRIEND

Meditating with a friend or loved one can open up your awareness to the special connection you have, or draw your attention to the other person's needs and how best you can support them. Try this exercise with someone you care about.

1. Sit facing your friend(s) on chairs or cushions. Together, settle into a quiet space. Let the silence remove any pressure or anxiety you may feel from your daily life. Try to accept yourself exactly as you are, and be released from fear, confusion and selfishness.

2. You may meditate in this way without words, but if you or anyone else present cares to, you can express aloud your experience. Try to receive what others say in a positive way, and look for the underlying truth.

3. Contemplate what is essential and eternal rather than trivial. If you speak, express yourself simply and with respect.

4. End your meditation session whenever your group feels ready.

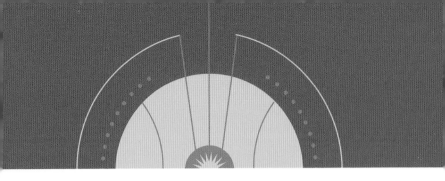

Journal prompt: Write a friendship affirmation

Genuine love manifests in different expressions, such as friendship, compassion, kindness, gratitude, appreciation, generosity and humility. Such love expresses itself freely. It is not defined through various conditions, not offered in exchange for something. Instead, it is revealed as an offering to life.

There is a wholeness to this love – it never creates divisions of 'for' and 'against', but instead seeks to express a unitive sense of things. Such love embraces the majestic sweep of existence without neglecting the ordinary and the everyday. The unstoppable force of friendship marks the sign of a mature and evolved human being.

In your journal, try to write out an affirmation of friendship and read it to yourself as a mediation on a regular basis.

There are examples on the next page.

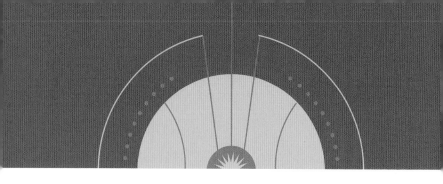

- May my mother and father live in peace and harmony.

- May my brothers and sisters live in peace and harmony.

- May my friends and neighbours live in peace and harmony.

- May the friendly, the strangers, and the unfriendly live in peace and harmony.

- May I live in peace and harmony.

- May my words and actions contribute to the happiness and welfare of others.

- May the power of my friendship transform difficult situations.

- May all beings live in peace and harmony.

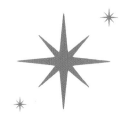

MINDFUL TALKING AND LISTENING

Communicating is one of the most important ways in which we build a sense of connection with those we care about. But when we are busy and distracted, the quality of our communication suffers. We cannot listen fully if we have one eye on a screen and one eye on our friend; we cannot respond adequately if we are trying to look something up online at the same time as talking to someone.

It all comes down to doing one thing at a time, as we discussed on page 36. Giving someone your complete and focused attention shows them that you value them, and enables you to feel truly connected.

The next time you have a conversation with a friend or loved one, make that the only thing you are doing. Put away your phone, turn off the TV. Perhaps even put down your knife and fork if you're at dinner, and try to give the other person your full attention. Listen to the words they're saying; give each sentence the focus it deserves. Observe their body language and facial expressions; listen to the words they aren't saying as well as those they are. Don't just wait for them to finish talking so that you can talk again – really listen and absorb. When it is time for you to respond, try to do so mindfully, thoughtfully, with compassion and care.

True friendship and connection is an incredibly special thing; give it the time and attention it deserves, and it will flourish.

EXPRESSING FRIENDSHIP

There are many ways in which you can choose to express love and compassion towards your friends or loved ones. By expressing your love and care to them in a mindful way, you may find that your connections and relationships with others go from strength to strength. Here are some ideas for ways in which you can mindfully express friendship and reinforce connection.

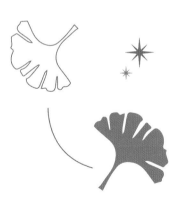

- Make small gestures of connection on a daily basis – send a simple message, invite someone out for a walk or a coffee, ask people for their opinions.

- At times, observe noble silence rather than engaging in negative reactivity.

- Listen to the kind voice within rather than the hard and harsh one.

- Wait at least twenty-four hours before sending a text or email that reveals anger.

- Step away from lingering resentment and into a space of compassion and patience.

- Develop a warmth and generosity of spirit rather than remaining stuck in old patterns.

- Remember to treat others as you wish to be treated.

EXPLORING CONNECTION WITH OTHERS

Examine your commitment to serve others, whether friends, family members or strangers. What practical steps can you take to support the needs of others and show them that you care?

Reflect on the difference between expressing love and compassion and holding on to notions of doing good. Truly compassionate actions are not performative acts of charity, but quiet and meaningful efforts to help and support others from a place of mutual care and respect.

If you are reasonably free from anguish and pain, and feel you have the strength and capacity within you to offer support and share that freedom with others, near or far, consider the ways in which you might be able to do that, whether it's through

✳

Make small gestures of connection on a daily basis.

✳

> **The greatest contribution to a good night's sleep is a relaxed attitude towards events during the day.**

volunteering for an organisation or simply making a cup of coffee for a friend or colleague who you know is having a challenging day.

At every moment, remember the great depth of interconnection we have with each other.

THE POWER OF KINDNESS

An essential part of our relationship to life is the expression of kindness.

We may think that we have a great deal of fear and anger to work on within ourselves, and we may feel as if that fear and anger are obstructing the free flow of kindness. Through developing the power of kindness, we can deconstruct the forces of fear and anger, loosening and lessening their grip on our existence.

Once we have convinced the heart and mind to truly develop kindness and friendship, and once we start truly putting it into practice, an inner power develops that becomes fearless. This expresses itself through the way we think, what we say and what we do.

Kindness is stronger than fear and anger.

KINDNESS TOWARDS OTHERS

Sometimes, it is easy to be kind; it just comes to us very naturally. At other times, judgements or our own problems can get in the way of our kindness. That's natural, too. But if we become more aware of our kindness, then it will blossom, reaching into those spaces of judgement and frustration, and helping us to overcome them. If we are willing, too, to become more aware of those times and spaces where we lack kindness – without being self-critical or loading ourselves up with guilt – then we also have the chance to dig out a few weeds.

Turning our kindness outwards and trying to extend it to others, even at times when we don't feel like it, can help us to feel more connected and present in our daily interactions, and help us find pleasure and joy in small moments that we might not usually consider significant.

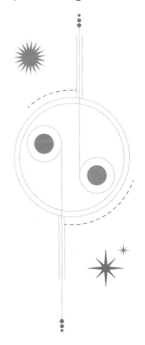

KINDNESS TOWARDS OURSELVES

Each of us is a remarkable and unique human being; each of us deserves kindness and compassion. Kindness should not just be directed outwards, however. It is something we should also try to direct inwards, by practising kindness towards ourselves.

This can be challenging; sometimes we are brought up to consider being kind to oneself as an act of selfishness or self-indulgence. However, practising self-kindness is actually a selfless act, as it nourishes and revives us, and ultimately gives us the strength and power to show up for others in a way we otherwise would not be able to.

It is all too easy to be self-critical or focus on our own flaws – it can certainly feel easier to do that than to be compassionate and loving towards ourselves. But the key to

Each of us is a remarkable and unique human being; each of us deserves kindness and compassion.

loving others is learning to love ourselves, just as we are. Use your mindfulness practice to help you begin treating yourself with the patience, compassion and kindness that you would show to a dear friend.

The next time you catch yourself beginning to self-criticise or dwelling on your perceived faults, try to shine the light of compassion on yourself instead. If you wouldn't say it to someone you cared about, don't say it to yourself.

How can you be kinder to yourself today? Can you give yourself the gift of time for meditation or quiet contemplation? Can you give yourself the gift of a nourishing meal, eaten mindfully, with every morsel relished? Can you give yourself the gift of setting aside your inner critic and instead celebrating your daily accomplishments?

How can you be a true friend to yourself?

Practising self-kindness is actually a selfless act, as it nourishes and revives us.

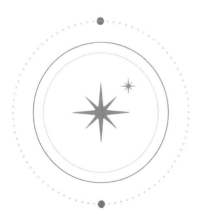

Meditating on kindness and friendship towards others acts as an important stepping stone on the path to compassion.

PRACTISING COMPASSION

It is not unusual to believe that compassion is something that we either have or don't have. Wisdom encourages us to develop and apply compassion, since it expresses wisdom about our relationship to the world. Meditating on kindness and friendship towards others acts as an important stepping stone on the path to compassion.

Some people in secular culture express a wise approach to daily life through their capacity to let go of issues, to regard them as a challenge and to live with passion. A spiritual approach to life goes further than this. It points to achieving an ultimate freedom through developing a deeply caring relationship with every area of existence.

Compassion towards others is an indispensable feature of mindful living.

Meditation, reflection, communication with others, acts of selfless service and wise use of resources are steps along the path to a noble way of living. It is an enormous challenge to adopt a compassionate view towards all forms of life on Earth. If we are not distracted by and charged up with ambition, the desire to make a name for ourselves or the need to become rich, we can live a life of service from one day to the next.

Compassion towards others is an indispensable feature of mindful living.

We can make a meaningful contribution towards the welfare of people, animals and the environment. Compassion is wisdom that directly benefits others. For generations, Buddhists have illustrated this with the image of a great bird flying through the air – one wing is for compassion and the other wing is for wisdom. If we apply both wings to our journey through existence, we abide in a meaningful and balanced way.

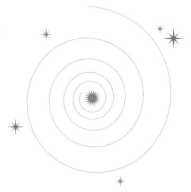

A MINDFUL APPROACH TO COMPASSION

We have become so infatuated with our thoughts – especially our memories and our plans, that we barely have enough headspace left to take an honest look at the present moment. There is no ultimate satisfaction to be found in this way of living, because it means our reality is made up of images, projections and stories.

Part of mindfulness practice consists of going beyond these stories about ourselves, about who we think we are, and what we think the world is like, and instead connecting with the real world and the intimacy of our relationship with it – here and now.

Taking a mindful approach to compassion and trying to incorporate it into everything we do can help us to achieve this connection.

Buddhist monk and Cambodian patriarch, Venerable Maha Ghosananda, used to remind people of a simple truth by saying:

The thought manifests as the word;

The word manifests as the deed;

The deed develops into the habit;

The habit hardens into the character;

The character gives birth to the destiny.

So, watch your thoughts with care,

And let them spring from love,

Born out of respect for all beings.

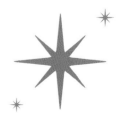

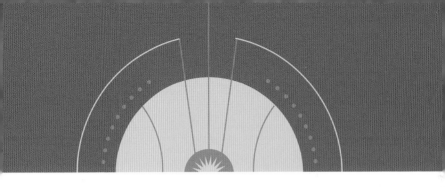

Journal prompt: What makes you feel connected?

As we approach the end of this chapter, spend some time making a list of all the situations, people and things that spark a feeling of connection within you, from reading a book that fires your imagination to gathering with friends at the beach, playing catch with your dog or walking through the trees. It could even be a fleeting moment, like making eye contact with someone on a train when something funny happens. It may seem obvious, but unless we consciously acknowledge these moments of connection, we will take them for granted, and so miss the opportunity to shape our lives so that we can feel more connection.

Feeling connected is an incredible source of grounding energy – it is extremely nourishing to our sense of self. So, take a few minutes to bathe in that energy as you list anything that helps you to feel connected, whether great or small. These moments give you an appreciation of life as it is, rather than as you feel it should be.

> A vital part of
> letting go is
> forgiveness, so
> ask yourself now:
> What or who
> do you need
> to forgive?

FORGIVENESS AND LETTING GO

The idea of letting go might seem counterintuitive when we're talking about the importance of connection, but sometimes we hold on to things that block the connections that are really essential. We might hold on to bad habits, old ideas about ourselves that no longer serve us, or feelings of anger or resentment towards others.

A vital part of letting go is forgiveness, so ask yourself now: What or who do you need to forgive?

If this question triggers a painful response, take your time. Bring your awareness to the feelings that have been brought up, and examine them if you feel able. If you feel that this is not the right moment, allow yourself the space to step away, and come back to the question when you feel ready.

It is a good idea to begin practising with small acts of forgiveness – letting go of little grievances that, in the grand scheme of things, don't really matter, especially in this present moment.

Writing down your forgiveness can be a powerful act, so you might choose to explore these experiences in your journal. How does it feel to forgive something? Notice your emotions; pay attention to what is happening in your body. You might feel a sense of relief or release, or you might feel that you don't actually mean it; that you're not ready to let go of this just yet. There is no pressure to forgive in this moment. There is no need to force your feelings. Simply accept and acknowledge the feelings that arise.

As you progress towards forgiving larger things, you may come across the sense that you need to forgive yourself. You might not even know exactly why or what for, but you may find you are carrying the old remnants of guilt with you. Ask yourself: where do you feel guilt in your body in this moment? Breathe into that place and the sensation you find there. Imagine breathing compassion into this place. As you do this, simply sit in awareness, observing but not attaching to any thoughts and feelings that come... and go.

There is no need to resolve the question of who or what you need to forgive in this moment; simply allow yourself to enquire and explore the thoughts or feelings that arise. Forgiveness can take time, but it is a radical act of compassion, both to yourself and to others, and you may find that letting go of the feelings you've been holding on to allows you more space for the things that truly matter.

A MINDFUL APPROACH TO EVERYDAY LIFE

Throughout this book, we have explored the idea of mindfulness in a way that ties in with real, normal life. It is easy to think of mindfulness as something that 'other people' do; we might have vague ideas of people wearing robes and lighting incense, and drifting about in a beautiful mountaintop temple with an air of serenity and calm. But mindfulness is for everyone, and each of us has the ability to tap into this incredible resource and begin to start appreciating and experiencing life with a level of richness we might never have thought possible.

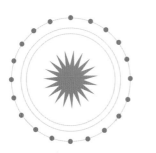

Forgiveness can take time, but it is a radical act of compassion.

From taking the time to appreciate tiny moments to slowly making changes that will have significant impacts on our wider lives, the practice of mindfulness creates a sense of calm, order, self-compassion and gentle curiosity that can be soothing and illuminating in equal measure.

Even on the busiest of days, allowing yourself a moment or two to stop, to breathe, to look around, to experience what is, can centre you and help you feel grounded, capable and at ease. It can also help you extend that sense of ease and calm to others; your friends, colleagues and family members will find you more comfortable and relaxing to be around, and you may find that your relationships become more harmonious as a result.

So, whenever you can – taste your food. Feel your feet on the ground. Run your fingers over your clothing. Listen wholeheartedly. Look at the clouds. Inhale the fragrance of coffee, perfume, flowers, clean laundry, fresh herbs, cut grass, spring rain. Find gratitude within yourself for the big things and the small things that make up the fabric of your world, and notice the endless network of connections that ties us all together with the universe.

Breathe.

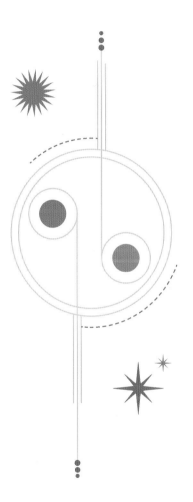

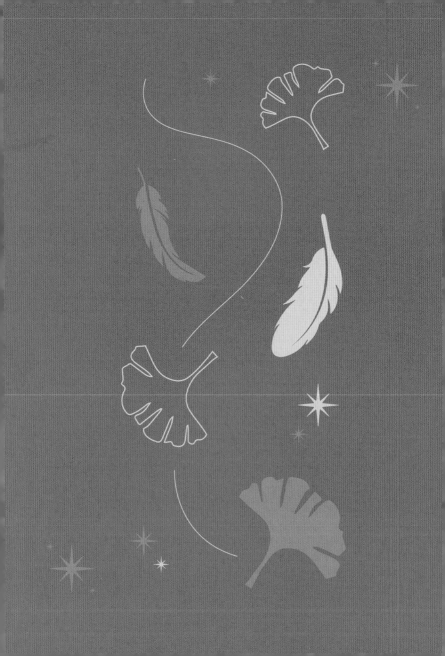